GEORGE MAYBERRY

Marijuana
and the
Volcano
Vaporization
System

Webster & Steele

Paperback ISBN: 978-0-578-23665-0

TABLE OF CONTENTS

1.

~~

INTRODUCTION

THIS LITTLE BOOK will describe a new method of smoking marijuana. I discovered this method a little more than ten years ago, and at that time I shared this information with a few friends. Some of them liked it very much and adopted it as their preferred way of smoking. Now, after ten years of using it, these friends are still enthusiastic about it and have made it the only way they smoke at home.

Some of my friends however did not care for this method for a variety of reasons: I like to take one really big hit and go on about my business; this way is too slow, I don't have the time; I don't like to have all the equipment needed if I smoked this way; yes, it is a better way to smoke, but I don't want to go to all that trouble to smoke; etc. As for expenses, I acknowledge that the price of the equipment needed is quite high, several hundred dollars.

Before we go further, I want to lay down a foundation for what we will be talking about.

There are basically two ways to smoke. One way is to ignite the herb so that it burns and throws off smoke. We are all familiar with this method. Tobacco and marijuana are smoked this way in pipes, in cigarettes, and in cigars. The second method of smoking is to heat the herb to a high temperature lower than the ignition temperature, at which point the herb starts emitting smoke.

This system was almost unknown in the West until recently, but was well known in Asia and the Middle East.

For example, in the Chinese opium pipe, the opium is never ignited. The pipe is constructed with a long stem of hollow bamboo. One end is the mouthpiece, the other end is sealed off. Near the closed end, an opening is cut to make a mounting for a ceramic bowl. The bowl is heated by an oil lamp and gets to be very hot. The prepared opium is dabbed onto it. The smoke produced is then sucked by the smoker through the bamboo stem.

A primitive way of smoking opium is to dab the opium onto the edge of an iron grillwork installed over an open fire. The smoker gets just above the opium, opens his mouth and breaths in as much of the smoke as he can.

This method of smoking is today called vaporization. Vaporization means that the smoke is not produced by burning but by high heat.

Beginning slowly in the 1960s, the development of vaporization and the availability of specialized equipment has been rapid. On the leading edge today, terms like hot, or very hot, are replaced by precise temperatures. Among the specialized equipment available today, the Volcano Vaporization System is among the leaders.

2.

~~~

The Volcano Family

To date there have been three models of the Volcano. All Volcanos are made by Storz & Bickel, an ethical German manufacturer of medical equipment. All three models work more or less the same way.

The Volcano itself is a "hot box". You plug it in and set the temperature you want and turn on the heater. The air inside the Volcano is heated until it reaches the temperature that was set. When the operator is ready to do so, he presses a button to start the motor pumping the hot air up through an opening at the top of the Volcano. The hot air goes up into the room. It does not get cooler because the heater turns itself on when the temperature of the entrapped air starts to decrease.

The next thing to talk about is the Filling Chamber. It is a short cylinder with a screen at the top and another screen at the bottom. Between these two screens, the operator will put the herb, say marijuana, and fit the Filling Chamber onto the top opening of the Volcano. Then, when the blower is turned on, hot air is forced through the Filling Chamber. Hot air goes in, smoke comes out. If nothing more is done, the smoke shoots up and starts to fill the room.

But something else is done. A balloon is attached to the top of the Filling Chamber so the smoke goes into the balloon. When the balloon is filled completely with smoke, the operator turns off the blower.

The balloon is detached and a mouthpiece is inserted into the bottom of the balloon. The smoker (who is usually the operator) can then smoke the marijuana.

The marijuana in the Filling Chamber can continue to give out more smoke, enough smoke to fill several balloons before this particular batch becomes exhausted.

This system of smoking was new, as far as I know, and created much discussion and much excitement.

The three different models of the Volcano. although somewhat similar, have differences, and we will now discuss these.

- The first model, now called the Volcano Classic, came out in 2000. It was fun to play with but I was a little disappointed. Repeated experiments gave different results. Something was unstable, and it was the temperature.

This machine is still being made, but I now regard it as a museum piece, very important historically, but completely surpassed by later models.

- The second model, called the Volcano Digit, came out in 2007. This model has good stable temperature control. Two days after I received this model, I knew there was something in my wild ideas that would pay off. After a couple of months experimenting, I was able to work out the details, and standardize the method of smoking I am about to explain.

Historically the Volcano Digit was the first machine that made it possible to smoke using this method. In 2019 Storz & Bickel discontinued making the Volcano Digit.

The last few years of its life, the Volcano Digit sold for $500. In addition, another $100 was needed for auxiliary equipment. That is to say, it cost $600 minimum to set up this mode.

- The third model, called the Volcano Hybrid, came out in 2019. It cost $700.

The Volcano Hybrid will do everything the Volcano Digit could do, and will heat to operating temperature much faster.

So much for the machines. Now I want to talk about the balloons. Storz & Bickel make pre-mounted balloons called the Easy-Valve Balloons. These come in two sizes: the 2-foot balloon and the 3-foot balloon. You want to use the 2-foot balloon. You do not want to use the 3-foot one. The reason for this will become apparent later. We will call the 2-foot balloon the standard balloon.

Storz & Bickel are also offering the option of letting the customer mount his own balloons. Don't do it! The work is tedious and frustrating and the end result is not really satisfactory. But I don't want to exclude anybody. If you decide to try self-mounting, see the Appendix: Mounting Balloons, p. 17.

3.

❧

GETTING READY TO SMOKE

I AM MORE or less assuming that you have either a Volcano Digit or a Volcano Hybrid and that you have more or less read the Owner's Manual that came with the Volcano.

I discuss things not in the Manual and also for emphasis some things that are.

- Use Fahrenheit

There are two modes on the Volcano, Fahrenheit and Celsius (formerly called Centigrade). Set it to the Fahrenheit mode. Why? Because then you have better control over the temperature.

Suppose you are in the Fahrenheit mode, and you want to increase the temperature a little. The smallest increase you can make is 1°F. If that's not enough, then 2°F, and so on. The settings must be in whole numbers, not fractions, and no decimal points.

If you are in Celsius mode, the smallest increase is 1°C. If that's not enough, then 2°C, etc. Now

1°C = 1.8°F, so 1°F is smaller than 1°C and so you can make finer adjustments.

To change from Fahrenheit to Celsius, or the other way around, look at the Volcano, you will see two buttons, one (+) for raising the set temperature, and the other (-) for lowering it. Press both buttons simultaneously: this is the toggle between Fahrenheit and Celsius mode.

• Loading marijuana.

You will put ground marijuana into the Filling Chamber. The amount you put in should not exceed the limit given in the Owner's Manual. My suggestion is that, if you are a beginner, get a set of kitchen measuring spoons, and put a half-teaspoon of marijuana into the Filling Chamber. This amount is equal to 2.5 ml (milliliters) or 2.5 cc (cubic centimeters).

I would suggest that you continue with this half-teaspoon amount any time you need to reload. After you get more experience you can put a larger amount if you want to.

• Pre-heating

To give out smoke, marijuana must be at a rather high temperature. When things start, hot air is flowing through marijuana that is at room temperature. But after a while the hot air heats the marijuana, and finally the marijuana has a temperature equal to that of the hot air and will produce smoke.

How long does this take? According to the Owner's Manual that comes with the Volcano it takes 5 seconds. This value, of course, is nominal. The time may vary somewhat, but to keep from going crazy trying to figure out the time, just use 5 seconds. That's close enough.

Now you attach the Filling Chamber to the Volcano. Do not attach a balloon to the Filling Chamber yet. When the blower starts, the hot air and some smoke flows through the Filling Chamber and goes out into the room. After 5 seconds have passed, attach the balloon to the Filling Chamber, and the smoke goes into the balloon. You do not turn off the blower during this process.

To carry out this process, you get the balloon ready. Maybe you should have a clock with a conspicuous second hand. You start the blower and then you have 5 seconds to get the balloon ready so that you can snap it down exactly 5 seconds after the blower started.

- Filling the balloon.

For reasons that will be explained later, the balloon should be fully inflated without letting any smoke escape into the room. It would seem fairly simple to fill the balloon, but beginners can mess it up.

You watch the balloon inflating and it begins to look like a cylinder with rounded ends, like a sausage. The rounded ends try to get square but never make it. Suddenly there is a rattling sound, a chattering sound, that can be quite loud. When you hear it, turn off the blower at once. Ideally you turn off the blower just before these noises start. With a little experience, you will get quite good at doing this. The chattering noises indicate that smoke is escaping the system and going out into the room. This hook-up is not meant to handle high pressure and the smoke leaks out in various places.

4.

~~

STARTING TO SMOKE

BEGIN WITH A virgin batch of marijuana in amount of, say, a half-teaspoon. What temperature should you begin with? Different people start with different temperatures, but these temperatures seem to be always between 300°F and 345°F.

Now I will give an ideal picture of what happens. Say you start at 330°F. When the Volcano has reached this temperature, pre-heat the marijuana for 5 seconds, then immediately attach the balloon and fill it. Then remove the Filling Chamber and the balloon. Put the Filling Chamber on a small plate (if you put it down on the table, you will probably get a dusting of marijuana on the table). Disconnect the balloon from the Filling Chamber and insert the mouthpiece into the bottom of the balloon.

The next step is very important and will require some discussion. You examine the smoke in the balloon and decide whether or not its density is satisfactory. What density is that? One that is not too much and not too little. In between is just right. The Goldilocks principle. The trouble with this description is that you don't know what density is just right. That is the case for everyone who learns this method, but after experience, the smoker learns how to recognize the right density.

If the density is correct, the smoke will be mild and smooth and won't cause coughing and also will have just the right amount of kick in it.

To do another extraction from this same sample of marijuana, raise the temperature 3°F, and make your second extraction. Once again, look at the density and verify that it is about right. Then, smoke the second balloon. It should also be mild and gentle with just the right amount of kick.

For another extraction, repeat the directions in the preceding paragraph. For each extra extraction, repeat the directions again. And again. And again.

You don't do all this at one sitting. When you feel you have had enough, you stop. You can start again the next day, or the next week, or whenever. It will take a number of extractions before the kick starts to disappear. When that happens, stop. Empty out and clean the Filling Chamber, and reload with another half-teaspoon of virgin marijuana, and start all over again at your beginning temperature.

This description is for an ideal smoking experience. How often will this happen? More than you might think. With an experienced smoker, most experiences work out very well. Does anything ever go wrong? Yes, it can. The density of the smoke tells what is going on. If the smoke starts to get a little too dense, it is still close to what it should be, you smoke that balloon. But for the next balloon, you make an adjustment. You raise the temperature only 2°F, and this will probably restore the next balloon to normal. After that, you return to 3°F and use that increase over and over again.

If the smoke does not have enough density, it will still be close enough that you can smoke that balloon, but then you increase the temperature by 4°F to restore the next balloon to normal. After that, you return to 3°F increases.

With these directions, you can begin smoking with this method.

By observing the density of the smoke tied together with your feelings about the smoke, you are on your way to master this method of smoking.

Why 3°F? Is 3 a magic number whose secret is revealed only by careful study of advanced numerology? No, it is not. What determines the use of 3°F is the volume of the standard balloon when it is filled completely.

5.

~~

OTHER SET-UPS

SUPPOSE WE WERE given a large balloon that had a volume exactly double that of the standard balloon. How would we handle that? Answer: we would raise the jump temperature to 6°F. We have to fill two standard balloons to get this volume, and each of them would require a 3°F raise, so 3°F + 3°F = 6°F is the amount the temperature rise would be.

Next, suppose we had a small balloon whose volume is exactly half of the full standard balloon. How would that be handled? Answer: we would raise the temperature by ½ ×3°F = 1.5°F between balloons. So we fill each half balloon and raise the temperature by 1.5°F between balloons. That is correct but there is just a little problem with our Volcanos, we can raise the temperature 1°F or 2°F but we cannot raise it 1.5°F.

So what can we do? Easy. Just raise the temperature by 2°F, then next time, by 1°F, then next time, 2°F and then 1°F, etc. In other words, 2, 1, 2, 1, 2, 1,.... The average rise would be 1.5°F, and we are home free. There is the inconvenience that we have to remember what the last rise was before we know the next rise.

For a final example, suppose that the Volcano had come with a balloon only 80% of our current standard balloon. This is roughly the same size, but the optimum jump would be 0.80 × 3°F = 2.4°F. How could we handle this? Jump back and forth between 2°F and 3°F and make adjustments when the smoke gets too dense or not dense enough. Very inconvenient. Did the manufacturer choose a balloon that had an optimum jump of 3°F? I feel certain that they did not. They determined the standard size using other criterion. So why does the standard size have this convenient jump of 3°F? Answer: pure luck.

Finally, we will discuss a particular example that might be of use to you. First consider a balloon of $2/3$ the size of the standard balloon. We don't actually need such a balloon because we will use a trick. Measure how many seconds it takes to fill the standard balloon. Say it is 34 seconds (if you measure this yourself, use your figure, not mine). Now $2/3$ × 34 seconds = 26.666... seconds (I used a calculator). We say 27 seconds is the fill time for the $2/3$ balloon, so we let the blower run this long then turn it off. It has pumped in the volume of a $2/3$ balloon. Now what is the optimum temperature jump for this quantity? Answer: $2/3$ ×3°F = 2°F. So, we will raise the temperature 2°F between balloons.

In practice, it is good to have a simple stop-watch. The blower will run 5 seconds for the warm-up, then another 27 seconds to "fill" the $2/3$ balloon. The blower will be running 5 + 27 = 32 seconds.

Now to smoke, you put the Filling Chamber on top of the Volcano, and get the balloon ready to snap onto the Filling Chamber after warm-up. When you turn on the blower for warm-up, you simultaneously start the stop-watch. You now have 5 seconds to get the balloon ready so that it can be attached the instant the stop-watch reads 5 seconds, then you wait until the stop-watch shows 32 seconds and turn off the blower. You know the rest.

Maybe after a few balloons you may find that the smoke is getting too dense. You can make a correction by increasing the fill time from 27 seconds to 28 seconds. That may be enough. If not continue to 29 seconds. Trial and error.

If the smoke is consistently becoming not dense enough, you lower the fill time from 27 to 26 or even 25 seconds.

This scheme can actually be useful: if you want a balloon not quite as big as the standard one, you can just use the $^2/_3$ balloon with the 2°F option.

The question can arise, is not this method of smoking wasteful? If you don't want to finish smoking a balloon, is not the remaining smoke discarded? How can this be justified?

My answer to this situation is this: I smoke to get the best smoke I can. I do not smoke to get the cheapest smoke I can.

6.

~~~

COMMENTS

THERE IS A rule so obvious that you seldom hear it said.

"Don't smoke marijuana when you don't want to."

Let us talk about a smoker, whose name is, say, Howard. Howard says he follows this rule always. Now let us look at Howard a little closer. He fills a balloon with smoke, and smokes all of it. He wants a bit more, so he fills a second balloon. After he smokes, say, ¼ of this second balloon, he has had all he really wants, so he stops. This is where the trouble begins. What does he do with that balloon which is ¾ filled with good smoke? There is no one else around who wants to smoke. It won't last until he wants to smoke again. It must be emptied because otherwise the smoke will all condense on the walls of the balloon. He can't stand the idea of wasting all that good smoke, so he finally decides to smoke and finish the balloon. Nothing has been wasted. Or has it? If it were all "wasted", there would be no harm done. Did he gain anything by smoking it himself? I would say no. What he did was harmful to him. He smoked more than he wanted to. Did he enjoy it? Again, I would say no. He was not smoking marijuana, marijuana was smoking him.

There are many Howards in this world. Some of them may be reading this book. If you don't see anything wrong with what Howard did, I would ask you to think about it some more.

Now I want to discuss smoking with other people. When the Volcano first appeared, it was too often a party device. Install a turkey bag, it makes a big balloon. It was used to pass around to all the people there, something like passing a joint down the line. I do not like to smoke that way.

If you go to a tea party, they don't have a big cup of tea being passed around. Each person has his own cup. If wine is served at a dinner, there is not a big glass of wine being passed around. Each person has his own glass. Why should it be any different with the Volcano? Each smoker should have his own balloon.

In a small group of smokers, usually one person acts as Volcano Master and refills empty balloons. If you are the host of such a gathering, you may well be the Volcano Master yourself. And, most important, if you are the host of any small gathering of smokers, I think you should make it known to all of them that no one should feel he has to empty his balloon. Any time you feel that you have had enough, simply stop and just leave your balloon as it is. In this way, no one would feel that he is making a bad impression on his host by not emptying his balloon.

I could go on and on, expressing my views, opinions, and my own personal feelings, but I think I have said enough. I know that I have nothing more to add to this little book. I have already written all the appendices, so what I am writing now is the end of my little book. I wish to bid farewell to you, dear Reader, and I do hope that what I have written will be of use to you.

7.

~~~

APPENDIX: MOUNTING BALLOONS

MOUNTING BALLOONS

I REPEAT MY preference to use balloons already mounted by the manufacturer. It is frustrating to mount the balloons yourself. But for those who decide to do it, I will describe what is involved.

The Owner's Manual says to cut off a section of the flat tube in amount of 19 up to 23 inches. The Manual then tells you how to mount this balloon. My directions differ. I say cut off a section of the flat tube to a length 29½ inches. The entire tube is 4 times as long, so you can get 4 such sections. Then mount one of these sections following the directions in the Owner's Manual. You will get a balloon that is longer than what we want, but you can reduce its length to exactly what we want because the balloon is already mounted.

The length of an empty balloon is this: the distance between where the balloon leaves its mounting base to where the knot stops the tip of the balloon. You grab the base in one hand and the tip of the balloon in the other, and pull the balloon straight. Measure this distance in inches, using a yardstick.

What is very important is that you want a balloon that has the same volume as a balloon mounted by the manufacturer. The length of an empty balloon mounted by the manufacturer is 21½ inches. The long balloon you mounted has a length more than 21½ inches. All you have to do now is to put a second tip ending at the right place, and cut off the old tip. You now have a balloon of the size needed for the method of smoking described in this little book.

VOLUME OF BALLOON

If you are given a balloon made in this same way (cylinder circumference of 62 cm), what is its volume? I will give you a formula that will tell you the volume of the filled balloon.

First, measure in inches the length of the empty balloon. Call the number you get E_{in}. Let the volume of the filled balloon be V_{cc} measured in cc (cubic centimeters) or, what is the same thing, in ml (milliliters). The relation between these two numbers (E_{in} and V_{cc}) is given by the formula

Equation 1 $V_{cc} = (E_{in} - 5.5) \times 777$

For the balloons mounted by the manufacturer, $E_{in} = 21.5$ inches. Put this value in Equation 1 and you get

$V_{cc} = (21.5 - 5.5) \times 777$

Use your calculator and you get

$V_{cc} = 12,432$ so the volume is

12,400 ml or 12.4 liters. This is equal to 759 cubic inches or 3.28 U.S. gallons.

Suppose you want to have a certain volume V_{cc}. What is the value of E_{in} that will give you that volume?

Using high-school algebra, and solving Equation 1 for E_{in} we get

Equation 2 $E_{in} = (V_{cc} \div 777) + 5.5$

Some people do not think in terms of cubic centimeters or

milliliters. They think in terms of tokes. How many tokes in a standard balloon? Whose tokes are we talking about? Tarzan of the Apes could empty the balloon in 2 tokes, but I am not Tarzan of the Apes. Neither are you. For me, 7 full tokes will empty the balloon.

8.

～～

APPENDIX: FLAT COLLARS

FLAT COLLARS

WHEN MORE THAN one kind of marijuana is being smoked, or when two or more smokers are using the same Volcano, we have to do something to avoid confusion. If there are several Filling Chambers on the table, we need to know which marijuana is in which Filling Chamber, and also at what temperature it was last smoked. This information needs to be written down and somehow attached to each Filling Chamber.

We will use very thin cardboard (with the thickness of an index card) and cut out a circular disc of diameter of 2 to 3 inches, and from the center of this disc a circular hole of about ¾ inches diameter will be cut out. This makes a flat hoop, or a flat ring, or what I like to call it, a flat collar. Now hold the collar just above the Filling Chamber and let it fall around the small tower that is sticking up. The collar falls, with the tower sticking up through the hole in the collar. The collar itself now lies flat surrounding the base of the tower.

Of course, when a Filling Chamber is being used, its collar comes off and should be replaced as soon as the Filling Chamber is free.

We will return with more directions on how to cut out these collars. We go now to an example of how these collars can be used.

Bill and Tony both smoke, but share a Volcano. Bill smokes Rose Dawn (RD) and Purple Twilight (PT). He takes a black felt-tip marker and writes RD on one collar, and PT on another, and puts these collars on the correct Filling Chambers. Tony smokes Kansas City (KC), and Gorilla Glue (GG), and Babies Nap (BN). He writes these initials with a red felt-tip pen on collars, and places each collar on the correct Filling Chamber. Note: black initials mean Bill while red initials mean Tony.

Now on each collar, three-digit numbers are written with a regular pen or pencil, and on each collar all but the last number are crossed out. The last number not crossed out is, say, 384. This means that this marijuana was last smoked at 384°F, and for the next smoke 3°F should be added to 384°F so that the next smoke will be at 387°F. Occasionally the last number will be a little different, say, 375+. The "plus" means that the smoker thought that the smoke was becoming too dense and that adjustment would be needed for the next smoke. So the smoker will add just 2°F, and start again at 377°F. After that, the jump will return to 3°F.

You know what is coming next. Occasionally the last number written will be, say, 361-. The "minus" sign means that etc., etc., etc.

HOW TO MAKE FLAT COLLARS

Making the first satisfactory collar may take more time than you expect. But once you have a good collar, you lay it down flat on the cardboard you are using and draw an outline with a pen or pencil. Then cut out this copy. If it is also satisfactory, then you label the first good one as the master. You can now go into production without need for a ruler or a compass.

Collars can be cut of paper, but it is much better to use a thin cardboard like an index card. These cards are available in 3×5 inches size and also in 4×6 inches size. White cards with ruling on one side are good. The ruling makes it clear which is the back side. You can also get card stock (110 lbs.) of size 8½×11 inches.

You can draw circles freehand if you want, but I prefer to use a compass to draw the circles. It is neater that way. Before you draw circles, you should put a conspicuous dot or cross on the cardboard to indicate the center of the circles. Now draw a circle of diameter 2 to 3 inches. The advantage of a bigger circle is that you have more space for writing. Then using the same center, draw another circle of diameter ¾ inches. This size is critical and your measurements may not be accurate. But this is a trial. If the inner circle does not fit, you will make another trial, until you get a good collar.

To cut out these circles, first cut out the big circle. From the rim of the big circle cut a straight line going to the center of the circles. This cut makes it easier to cut out the inner circle. The cut can be left there, but if it bothers you, put a small piece of Scotch Tape on the backside to hold it together.

9.

~~

Appendix: Portable Vaporizers

Portable Vaporizers

Most of my friends who use the Volcano have chosen to also own a portable vaporizer. Their choice and mine, from the multitude of such instruments, is a little machine called the Mighty. It is made by Storz & Bickel and costs (2020) \$350. It has a shape sort of like a little box, measuring (in inches):

$H \times W \times D = 5\frac{1}{2} \times 3 \times 1\frac{1}{8}$.

It is not a match for the Volcano, but what else is? I think that the smoker needs at least two of them so that there is always one to smoke while the other is being recharged.

I would not give the Mighty to just anyone and say figure it out for yourself. They probably could not. But someone who has understood the way of smoking described in this little book would be able to figure it out for himself. Such a person knows the rule, start low and climb slow. How low is low? How slow is slow? Find out for yourself!

The major point of complaint about the Mighty is what we call the top, or cooling head. Smoke goes into it and comes out. The cooling function works well. The problem is that it gets dirty, and after a while the smoke takes on a bad taste, and the instrument itself starts to smell like an old pipe that needs cleaning. You can buy 3 extra tops for $56 (2020). Of course you still have to clean the tops.

It is difficult to do this cleaning. I know of people who used the Mighty and liked it, but stopped using it because it is easier to stop using it than it is to clean it.

Cleaning requires that you dis-assemble the stuff in the top. At first it looks very difficult, but after forcing yourself to do it a few times, it is not so bad. But cleaning all the parts is also difficult. First you can soak the parts in hot water with a good detergent. An hour or more for this. Then you have to clean (or try to clean) the parts by hand using brushes and other aids. After that, a soak in 95% ethyl alcohol may help.

There is a way to simplify the cleaning by using an ultrasonic (vibrating) machine. I asked one of my smoking friends to hunt for a good, cheap one, and she found it: a small one for $40 that does the job. With this system, the actual cleaning is much easier. After dis-assemblage, you put the dirty parts into the ultrasonic machine with hot water fortified with detergent, and let it vibrate for 30 minutes. Remove the parts. They don't look clean, but simply go over the surfaces lightly (no scrubbing) with a facial tissue or a Q-tip, and all the dirt comes off, and all the parts are clean.

The ultrasonic machine can be used for many other things. In particular, we clean the Filling Chambers that go with the Volcano.

www.ingramcontent.com/pod-product-compliance
Lightning Source LLC
Chambersburg PA
CBHW060532280326
41933CB00014B/3145